The Fast

Diet Cookbook for

Busy People

Quick and easy Alkaline Recipes to improve your Health and boost your Brain

Sam Carter

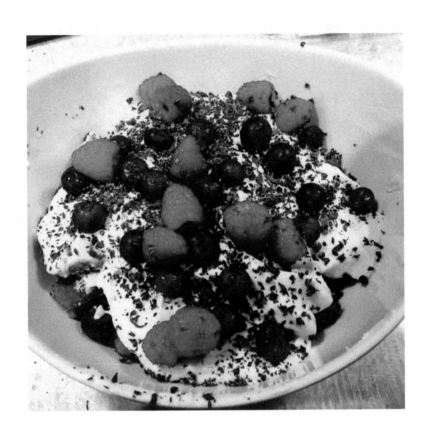

By reading this document, the reader agrees that under no circumstances is the author responsible for any losses, direct or indirect, which are incurred as a result of the use of information contained within this document, including, but not limited to, — errors, omissions, or inaccuracies.

Table of Contents

Chilled Tomato Soup

Servings: 2

Total Time: 10 minutes plus 2 hours chill time

Ingredients

- 3 tomatoes, peeled
- ½ large green bell pepper, finely chopped
- 1 ½ tablespoons apple cider vinegar
- 1 ½ tablespoons lemon juice
- 1 ½ cucumber, peeled, seeded and finely diced
- 2 shallots, sliced
- 1 jalapeno, seeded and diced
- 1 teaspoon cumin
- 1 teaspoon tamari
- 1 tablespoon olive oil
- 1 ½ tablespoons fresh parsley, chopped
- 1 tablespoon
- 1 teaspoon sugar free hot sauce

Directions

1.   Place all ingredients in a blend and combine until full mixed (mixture will not be entirely smooth). If a thinner soup is desired, add 1 tablespoon of water at a time until desired consistency is achieved.

2.   Chill in the fridge for 2 hours before serving.

Sweet & Sour Cabbage

Servings: 2

Total Time: 45 minutes

Ingredients

- 1 teaspoon ghee
- 1 teaspoon olive oil
- 1 shallot, thinly sliced
- ½ green cabbage, shredded
- ½ red cabbage, shredded
- 2 tablespoons raw honey
- ½ cup apple cider vinegar
- 1/3 cup water
- 1 teaspoon Himalayan salt
- 1 teaspoon black pepper, crushed
- ½ teaspoon nutmeg
- 1 tablespoon caraway seeds

Directions

1.   In a large pot, heat ghee and olive oil over medium heat and add the shallot, green and red cabbage. Cook for 10 minutes or until softened and coated with the oil and ghee.

2.   Add honey, vinegar, water, salt, pepper and nutmeg. Cook another 5 minutes then reduce heat to low and simmer for 30 minutes or until cabbage is soft.

3.   Stir in caraway seeds and serve warm.

Vegetable & Lentil Soup

Servings: 2

Total Time: 1 hour

Ingredients

- ½ tablespoon olive oil

- 1 garlic clove, minced

- ¼ cup carrots, diced

- ¼ cup celery, diced

- ¼ cup yellow onion, diced

- 1 small leek, white part sliced into half-moons and cleaned well

- ½ cup brown lentils, washed and drained

- 1 teaspoon dried rosemary

- 1 teaspoon dried thyme

- 2 cups water

- 1 tablespoon tomato paste

- 1 tablespoon apple cider vinegar

- 1 teaspoon Himalayan salt

- 1 teaspoon black pepper, crushed

- Handful spinach leaves

Directions

1.   In a large pot, olive oil and add garlic, onion, carrot, celery and onion. After 5 minutes add the leeks and cook an additional 10 minutes.

2.   Add the lentils, rosemary, thyme, water, tomato paste and vinegar. Cook, uncovered, for 45 minutes or until lentils are tender. Stir in spinach leaves and season with salt and pepper before serving.

Roasted Red Pepper Dip

Servings: 2

Total Time: 5 minutes

Ingredients

- 2 whole roasted peppers
- ¾ cup walnuts, toasted
- ½ cup green onions, sliced
- 2 garlic cloves
- ½ teaspoon Himalayan salt
- 1 tablespoon lemon juice
- 2 teaspoons raw honey
- 1 teaspoon ground cumin
- 1 teaspoon red chili flakes
- ½ teaspoon cayenne pepper
- ½ teaspoon red pepper flakes
- 3 tablespoons almond meal
- 4 tablespoons olive oil

Directions

1.   In a blender or food processor, combine all ingredients except leave a remaining 2 tablespoons of the olive oil.

2.   Blend until smooth and transfer to serving bowl. Stir in the remaining 2 tablespoons of olive oil.

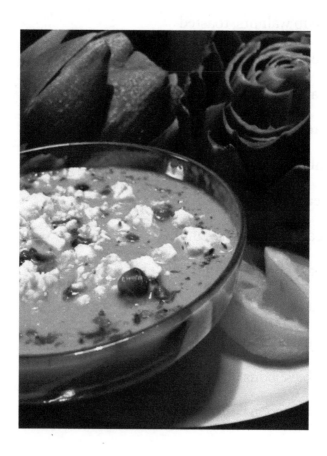

Ghee & Maple Roasted Carrots

Servings: 2

Total Time: 35 minutes

Ingredients

- 3 large carrots, washed and cut into 1 inch pieces

- 1 tablespoon ghee, melted

- 1 tablespoon maple syrup

- 1 teaspoon lemon zest

- 1 teaspoon Himalayan salt

- ¼ teaspoon black pepper, crushed

- 1 tablespoon sesame seeds, toasted

Directions

1. Preheat oven to 400°F/205°C.

2. In a small bowl, whisk together the ghee, maple syrup, lemon zest, salt and pepper.

3. Place carrots in a shallow baking dish and coat with ghee and maple mixture. Roast 25 minutes, turning once halfway through.

4.   Remove carrots from oven and sprinkle the sesame seeds.

Edamame Salad

Servings: 2

Total Time: 20 minutes

Ingredients

- 1 cup edamame, shelled, cooked and cooled
- 2 tablespoons green onions, sliced
- 1 cup cucumber, diced
- ¼ cup red onion, diced
- 1 teaspoon avocado oil
- 1 teaspoon sesame oil
- ½ teaspoon Himalayan salt
- ¼ teaspoon red chili flakes

Directions

1.   Toss all ingredients in a medium bowl and make sure it is all well coated.

2.   Chill in the fridge for 15 minutes before serving.

Smokey Caesar Salad

Servings: 2

Total Time: 15 minutes

Ingredients

- 1 large bunch kale, stems removes and thinly sliced
- 1 cup pumpkin seeds
- 5 cherry tomatoes, halved
- ½ cucumber, diced
- 1/3 cup almonds
- ⅛ teaspoon chipotle powder
- ½ teaspoon smoked paprika
- 2 garlic cloves
- 1 tablespoon nutritional yeast
- 1 ¼ cup filtered water
- 1 teaspoon honey
- ½ teaspoon Himalayan salt

Directions

1.   In a blender combine the almonds, chipotle powder, smoked paprika, garlic, nutritional yeast, water, honey and salt.

2.   Place kale, pumpkin seeds, cherry tomatoes and cucumber in a large bowl and cover with dressing mix from the blender.

3.   Toss well to ensure all the leaves are coated and let sit a few minutes before serving.

Baked Sweet Potato Fries with Spicy BBQ Sauce

Servings: 2

Total Time: 35 minutes

Ingredients

- 1 large sweet potato, cut into large julienne sticks
- 1 tablespoon avocado oil
- ½ teaspoon Himalayan salt
- ½ teaspoon garlic powder

Spicy BBQ Sauce

- 2 tablespoons tomato paste
- 1 tablespoon water
- 1 tablespoon maple syrup
- 1 tablespoon coconut aminos
- 1 teaspoon tamari
- 1 teaspoon smoked paprika
- 1 teaspoon chili powder
- ½ teaspoon cayenne pepper

Directions

1.   Make Spicy BBQ Sauce by combining all the Spicy BBQ Sauce ingredients in a blender.

2.   Preheat oven to 400°F/205°C. In a large bowl, toss sweet potato with oil, salt and garlic powder.

3.   Place sweet potato on one layer of parchment paper lined on a baking tray. Bake 20 minutes, flipping halfway through.

4.   Serve sweet potato fries with the Spicy BBQ Sauce.

Citrus & Jicama Salad

Servings: 2

Total Time: 35 minutes

Ingredients

- 1 orange, peeled and cut into bite-sized pieces
- 1 grapefruit, peeled and cut into bite sized pieces
- 1 jicama, shredded
- 3 cups spinach
- 3 tablespoons green onions, thinly sliced
- ½ head radicchio, thinly sliced
- 2 tablespoons olive oil
- 2 tablespoons orange juice
- 1 tablespoon lemon juice
- 1 teaspoon lemon zest
- ¼ teaspoon Himalayan salt
- ⅛ teaspoon ground cloves
- ⅛ teaspoon black pepper, crushed

Directions

1.   In a large bowl, combine orange pieces, grapefruit pieces, shredded jicama, spinach, green onions and radicchio.

2.   Whisk together the olive oil, orange juice, lemon juice, lemon zest, salt, ground cloves and black pepper in a small bowl to form the dressing.

3.   Pour dressing over the citrus and jicama salad and serve.

Green Cabbage Slaw

Servings: 2

Total Time: 15 minutes

Ingredients

- 1 avocado

- 3 tablespoons olive oil

- 1 lemon, juiced

- 1 teaspoon apple cider vinegar

- ¼ teaspoon Himalayan salt

- ½ cup green cabbage, thinly shredded

- 2 carrots, shredded

- 2 shallots, thinly sliced

- 3 tablespoons cilantro, finely chopped

- 1 tablespoon green onions, thinly sliced

- 1 tablespoon raisins

Directions

1.   Place avocado, olive oil, lemon juice, vinegar and salt in a blender and combine until smooth.

2.   In a large bowl combine the avocado mixture, cabbage, carrots, shallots, cilantro, green onion and raisins.

3.   Chill 10 minutes before serving.

Spicy Mix with Tortilla Chips

Servings: 2

Total Time: 5 minutes plus 30 minutes chill time

Ingredients

- 3 tomatoes, finely diced
- 1 green bell pepper, seeded and finely diced
- 2 green onions, thinly sliced
- 2 garlic cloves, grated
- 1 jalapeno, seeded and finely diced
- 2 tablespoons cilantro, finely chopped
- ½ teaspoon Himalayan salt
- ½ teaspoon cayenne pepper
- ¼ teaspoon red chili flakes
- 1 lime, juiced
- 1 tablespoon olive oil
- 24 sprouted corn tortilla chips

Directions

1.   In a medium bowl combine all the ingredients except the tortilla chips. Place half of the mixture in a blender or food processor and pulse 10 times.

2.   Add blended mix back to the bowl with the rest of ingredients and stir to combine.

3.   Chill at least 30 minutes before serving with tortilla chips.

Meatless Taco Wraps

Servings: 2

Total Time: 20 minutes

Ingredients

- 1 ½ cups brown lentils, cooked

- ½ cup walnuts, toasted

- 1 tablespoon tomato paste

- 1 garlic clove, minced

- ½ teaspoon smoked paprika

- ½ teaspoon chili powder

- ½ teaspoon cumin

- ½ teaspoon Himalayan salt

- ¼ cup water

- 4 romaine leaves

- ½ avocado, sliced

Rainbow Salsa

- ½ cup mango, diced

- ½ cup red bell pepper, diced

- ½ cup green bell pepper, diced

- 3 tablespoons cilantro, chopped

- 1 tablespoon apple cider vinegar

- ½ teaspoon Himalayan salt

- ½ teaspoon black pepper, crushed

Directions

1. Make Rainbow Salsa by placing all Rainbow Salsa ingredients in a medium bowl and stirring to combine. Let sit for 10 minutes while you make the taco meat.

2. In a food processor, pulse together the lentils, walnuts, tomato paste, garlic, paprika, chili powder, cumin, salt and water. The mixture should be crumbly and not overly smooth.

3. Place the lentil & walnut mixture into each of the romaine leaves and top with Rainbow Salsa and avocado slices.

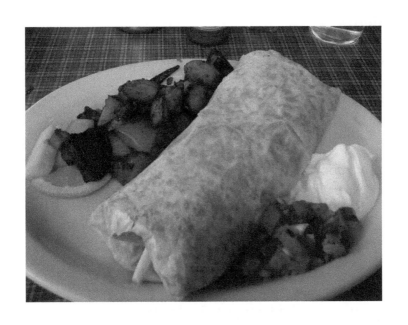

Quinoa & Black Sesame Pilaf

Servings: 2

Total Time: 25 minutes

Ingredients

- 1 cup green beans, trimmed and cut into 1 inch pieces
- 2 carrots, peeled and sliced into matchsticks
- 2 tablespoons olive oil, divided
- 2 teaspoons Himalayan salt, divided
- 2 teaspoons black pepper, crushed and divided
- 1 shallot, sliced
- 1 celery stalk, finely diced
- ½ cup green bell pepper, finely diced
- 1 garlic clove, minced
- ½ cup quinoa
- 1 cup vegetable broth or water
- 1 cup green lentils, cooked

Dressing

- 1/3 cup avocado oil

- 2 teaspoons toasted sesame oil

- 1 teaspoon fresh ginger, grated

- 1 teaspoon lemon zest

- ½ teaspoon red chili flakes

- ¼ cup tamari

- ¼ cup rice vinegar

- 2 tablespoons black sesame seeds, toasted

Directions

1. Place green beans and carrots on a parchment paper lined baking tray and drizzle with 1 tablespoon of olive oil, 1 teaspoon salt and 1 teaspoon black pepper. Cook under the broiler for about 5 minutes or until browned, turning about halfway through.

2. In a large pot, add remaining 1 tablespoon olive oil, shallot, celery, bell pepper and garlic, cooking for 5 minutes. Add quinoa, stirring to coat and cook 2 minutes, until toasted. Add broth or water, bring to a boil and then reduce heat and let simmer for 5 - 8 minutes or until liquid is absorbed.

3. To make dressing, add all dressing ingredients to a bowl and whisk to combine.

4. To assemble, mix together the lentils and quinoa. Season with remaining 1 teaspoon salt and 1 teaspoon pepper. Top with

green bean and carrot mixture before drizzling dressing over entire dish.

Lemon Zucchini Pasta

Servings: 2

Total Time: 15 minutes

Ingredients

- 4 zucchinis
- 2 cups baby spinach, roughly chopped
- 1 cup kale, stems removed and roughly chopped
- ¼ cup fresh basil
- ¼ cup parsley
- 3 garlic cloves
- 1 lemon, juiced
- ¼ cup cashews, soaked overnight and drained
- 2 teaspoons red chili flakes
- 2 teaspoons lemon zest
- 1 cup olive oil
- 1 teaspoon Himalayan salt
- 1 teaspoon black pepper, crushed
- ½ cup cherry tomatoes, sliced in half
- ¼ cup pine nuts, toasted

Directions

1.   Using a spiralizer (or a vegetable peeler to make wider noodles), make zucchini into noodles and set aside.

2.   In a food processor combine the spinach, kale, basil, parsley, garlic, lemon juice, cashews, red chili flakes and lemon zest. Once finely chopped, slowly drizzle in olive oil.

3.   In a large bowl, toss together the zucchini noodles with the spinach/kale sauce. Season with salt and pepper before garnishing with tomatoes and pine nuts.

Sweet Potato Stew

Servings: 2

Total Time: 50 minutes

Ingredients

- 1 tablespoon olive oil

- ½ yellow onion, diced

- 2 garlic cloves, minced

- 1 tablespoon tomato paste

- 1 tablespoon apple cider vinegar

- ¼ cup rice flour

- 2 cups vegetable broth

- 1 tablespoon tamari

- 1 tablespoon coconut aminos

- 1 large carrot, cut into 1 inch pieces

- 1 cup sweet potatoes, cut into 1 inch chunks

- 1 stalk of celery, cut into ½ inch pieces

- 1 cup green peas, defrosted if frozen

- ½ tomato, diced

- 1 bay leaf

- 1 teaspoon black pepper

- 1 teaspoon dried thyme

- 1 teaspoon oregano

- ¼ cup parsley, chopped

Directions

1.   Heat oil in a large pot over medium heat. Add onion and garlic and cook for 5 minutes. Add tomato paste, vinegar and rice flour. Stir the mixture with a spoon consistently for 5 more minutes.

2.   Pour in broth, tamari and aminos and add carrot, sweet potato, celery, peas, tomato, bay leaf, pepper, thyme and oregano.

3.   Let come to a boil and then reduce heat to low and simmer for 20 minutes.

4.   After 10 minutes, stir in parsley and serve.

Cashew Zoodles

Servings: 2

Total Time: 30 minutes

Ingredients

- 1 small zucchini, cut into noodles with a spiralizer
- 1 yellow squash, cut into noodles with a spiralizer
- 1 ¼ teaspoon Himalayan salt
- 2 cups cashews, soaked overnight and drained
- 1 lemon, juiced
- 3 tablespoons water
- 2 tablespoons olive oil
- ¼ teaspoon turmeric
- 1 garlic clove
- 1 teaspoon onion powder
- 2 tablespoons nutritional yeast
- 1 teaspoon black pepper
- 10 cherry tomatoes, halved
- 2 teaspoons chives

Raw Berry Crumble

Servings: 2

Total Time: 30 minutes

Ingredients

- 1/3 cup blueberries
- 1/3 cup blackberries
- 1/3 cup raspberries
- ½ cup mixed berries
- 2 dates, pitted, soaked 15 minutes and drained
- 2 teaspoons lime juice
- ¼ teaspoon Himalayan salt
- ¼ teaspoon vanilla extract

Crumble

- ½ cup pecans
- ½ cup walnuts
- ½ cup dates, pitted, soaked 2-4 hours and drained
- ¼ cup dried coconut
- 1 teaspoon cinnamon
- ¼ teaspoon nutmeg

- ¼ teaspoon Himalayan salt

Whipped Coconut Cream (optional)

- 1 can full fat coconut milk, chilled overnight in the fridge

- ½ teaspoon vanilla extract

- ½ teaspoon lemon zest

- 1 tablespoon maple syrup

Directions

1. Place the blueberries, blackberries and raspberries (excluding the ½ cup mixed berries) in a food processor with the dates, lime juice, salt and vanilla extract. Blend until combined well.

2. Toss together fruit mixture with remaining ½ cup of mixed berries in a small bowl. Spread mixture on the bottom of a small glass dish.

3. Clean the food processor and add all the Crumble ingredients to the food processor. Pulse to combine and stop when mixture is desired crumbly texture.

4. Crumble nut mixture over the fruit mixture.

5. If using the Whipped Coconut Cream, open the can of coconut milk and drain the water for later use. Add coconut cream to a bowl (preferably a chilled metal bowl) and add the

vanilla, lemon zest and maple syrup. Beat with a hand mixer for 3 minutes or until fluffy. Spoon on top of the crumble.

Coco-nutty Cookies

Servings: Makes 8 cookies

Total Time: 15 minutes plus 2 hours chilling

Ingredients

- 1 cup walnuts
- 1 ½ cup almonds
- 1/3 cup dates, pitted, soaked 15 minutes and
- 2 tablespoons raisins, soaked 15 minutes and drained
- ½ teaspoon almond extract
- ¼ teaspoon vanilla extract
- ¼ teaspoon Himalayan salt
- 2 tablespoons water
- ¼ cup unsweetened, shredded coconut

Directions

1. Combine all ingredients except the shredded coconut in a food processor until combined but not entirely smooth.

2. Roll dough into tablespoon sized balls. Roll each ball in shredded coconut and place on baking tray lined in parchment paper.

3.   Press each ball down slightly to form a cookie shape. Allow to chill for at least 2 hours before serving.

Chocolate Coconut Bites

Servings: Makes 12 bites

Total Time: 25 minutes plus 1 hour 30 minutes chill time

Ingredients

- ¾ cup (+1 extra tablespoon) finely shredded, unsweetened coconut, divided

- ¼ cup dates, pitted

- 1 tablespoon pecan butter

- 1 tablespoon cacao powder

- ¼ teaspoon Himalayan salt

- ¼ teaspoon vanilla

- 2 tablespoons pecans, crushed

Chocolate Coating

- 3 tablespoons cacao powder

- 3 tablespoons cacao butter, melted

- 1 tablespoon maple syrup

- ¼ teaspoon vanilla extract

- ½ teaspoon Himalayan salt

- Pinch Himalayan salt

Directions

1.   In a food processor, combine ½ cup of the shredded coconut, the dates and pecan butter. Combine until smooth. Add in ¼ coconut, cacao powder, salt and vanilla. Process until a ball of dough forms.

2.   Remove dough and shape into 6 balls. Place on a baking tray lined with parchment paper and chill 1 hour in the fridge.

3.   After 1 hour, prepare chocolate coating by whisking all the Chocolate Coating ingredients together in a small bowl.

4.   Remove chocolate coconut balls from the fridge. On a small plate, combine the pecans and 1 tablespoon shredded coconut. Dip each ball into the chocolate mixture, coating half of the ball and then dipping the chocolate coating in the pecan coconut mixture. Place back on the baking tray and chill again at least 30 minutes before serving.

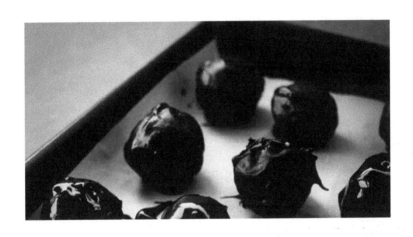

Squash Pudding Parfaits

Servings: 2

Total Time: 30 minutes

Ingredients

- ½ cup cashews, soaked overnight and drained
- ¼ cup pumpkin puree
- ¼ cup butternut squash puree
- ¼ teaspoon ground cinnamon
- ⅛ teaspoon ground nutmeg
- ⅛ teaspoon ground ginger
- ⅛ teaspoon Himalayan salt
- ⅛ teaspoon allspice
- 1 tablespoon maple syrup
- ¼ cup unsweetened almond milk
- 2 teaspoons melted coconut oil

Whipped Coconut Cream

- 1 can full fat coconut milk, chilled overnight in the fridge (Do not use Lite Coconut Milk)
- ½ teaspoon vanilla extract

- ¼ teaspoon cinnamon

- 1 tablespoon maple syrup

Pumpkin Pecan Praline (Optional)

- 2 tablespoons water

- 4 tablespoons coconut sugar

- ½ teaspoon Himalayan salt

- 2 tablespoons pumpkin seeds

- 2 tablespoons pecans, crushed

Directions

1. In a food processor, combine the cashews and the next 10 ingredients. Combine until smooth and set in fridge.

2. To make the Whipped Coconut Cream, open the can of coconut milk and drain the water for later use. Add coconut milk to a bowl (preferably a chilled metal bowl) and add the vanilla, cinnamon and maple syrup. Beat with a hand mixer for 3 minutes or until fluffy.

3. If using the Pumpkin Pecan Praline, line a baking tray with parchment paper. In a small saucepan over medium-high heat, add water and sugar. Stir to dissolve and let cook about 5 minutes being cautious not to burn. Add salt, pumpkin seeds and pecans,

stirring constantly. Pour mixture out onto baking tray. When completely cooled, break into pieces.

4.   In small jars, layer the squash pudding, whipped coconut cream and pumpkin pecan praline to serve.

Raspberry Cheesecakes

Servings: Makes 8 tarts

Total Time: 30 minutes

Ingredients

- ½ cup raw almonds
- ¾ cup dates, pitted and soaked for 15 minutes
- 1 teaspoon nutmeg
- 1 teaspoon cinnamon
- ½ teaspoon Himalayan salt
- 8 raspberries

Raspberry Cheesecake Filling

- ½ cup raw cashews, soaked for 1 hour and drained
- 3 tablespoons lemon juice
- ½ tablespoon lemon zest
- 3 tablespoons water
- ½ cup raspberries
- 1 teaspoon vanilla extract
- ¼ teaspoon almond extract
- 1 teaspoon raw honey

- ½ teaspoon Himalayan salt

Directions

1.   Make tarts shell dough by combining the almonds, dates, nutmeg, cinnamon and salt in a food processor. Pulse until mixture becomes crumbly then continue to blend until a slightly sticky ball form.

2.   Remove tart shell dough from food processor and form into 8 equal sized balls. Press each ball into a mini muffin or tart pan, making sure to create equal sides. Place pan in fridge for 10 minutes and then remove the shells.

3.   In a clean food processor, combine the Raspberry Cheesecake Filling ingredients until smooth.

4.   In each tart shell, add the Raspberry Cheesecake Filling and top with a raspberry.

Double Chocolate Mint Tarts

Servings: Makes 8 tarts

Total Time: 30 minutes

Ingredients

- ½ cup raw almonds
- ¾ cup dates, pitted, soaked and drained for 15 minutes
- 2 tablespoons raw cacao powder
- ½ teaspoon Himalayan salt
- 1 tablespoon cacao nibs
- 8 small mint leaves

Chocolate Mint Filling

- ½ cup raw cashews, soaked for 1 hour and drained
- 3 tablespoons water
- 1 teaspoon vanilla extract
- ¼ teaspoon mint extract
- 1 tablespoon maple syrup
- ½ teaspoon Himalayan salt

Directions

1.   Make tarts shell dough by combining the almonds, drained dates, cacao powder and salt in a food processor. Pulse until mixture becomes crumbly then continue to blend until a slightly sticky ball forms.

2.   Remove tart shell dough from food processor and form into 8 equal sized balls. Press each ball into a mini muffin or tart pan, making sure to create equal sides. Place pan in fridge for 10 minutes and then remove the shells.

3.   In a clean food processor, combine the Chocolate Mint Filling ingredients until smooth.

4.   In each tart shell, add the Chocolate Mint Filling and top with cacao nibs and mint leaves.

Brown Rice Pudding

Servings: 2

Total Time: 25 minutes

Ingredients

- 1 teaspoon ghee
- 2 tablespoons raisins
- 1 ½ cups brown rice, cooked
- 2 cups unsweetened almond milk
- 1 teaspoon cinnamon
- ½ teaspoon nutmeg
- ¼ teaspoon cloves
- 1 tablespoon maple syrup
- ¼ teaspoon Himalayan salt
- 1 tablespoon unsweetened, shredded coconut

Directions

1. Heat ghee in a small saucepan over medium-heat. Add raisins, brown rice, almond milk, cinnamon, nutmeg, cloves, maple syrup and salt.

2. Bring to a boil then reduce heat to low and simmer for 15 minutes or until liquid is absorbed.

3. Garnish with coconut and serve.

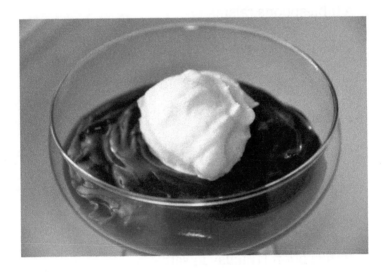

Baked Apples with Peanut Butter Sauce

Servings: 2

Total Time: 25 minutes

Ingredients

- 1 apple, cored and sliced into ½ inch slices
- 1 teaspoon coconut oil, melted
- 1 teaspoon cinnamon
- ½ teaspoon nutmeg
- ¼ teaspoon Himalayan salt
- ¼ teaspoon coconut sugar
- 2 tablespoons walnuts, crushed and toasted

Peanut Butter Sauce

- ¾ cup unsweetened yogurt
- 2 tablespoons peanut butter, melted
- ½ teaspoon cinnamon

Directions

1.	Preheat oven to 375°F/190°C. In a glass baking dish, layer the apple slices so they are slightly overlapping. Pour melted coconut oil over the top and sprinkle with cinnamon, nutmeg, salt and coconut sugar.

2.   Place baking dish in the oven and cook for 10 - 15 minutes.

3.   In a small bowl, mix together yogurt, peanut butter and cinnamon to create the Peanut Butter Sauce.

4.   Remove apples from the oven, drizzle the Peanut Butter Sauce on top and then add walnuts.

Fig Bites

Servings: Makes approx. 12 bites

Total Time: 20 minutes plus 2 hours chill time

Ingredients

- ½ cup dates, pitted
- ¼ cup raisins
- ¼ cup dried cherries
- ¼ cup figs
- ½ cup almond flour
- 1 teaspoon vanilla extract
- ¼ teaspoon Himalayan salt
- ¼ cup unsweetened, shredded coconut

Directions

1.   In a food processor combine dates, raisin, cherries and figs. Once well combined, begin adding the almond flour. Lastly, add vanilla and salt. Continue to process until a ball of dough forms.

2.   Place shredded coconut on a plate. Line a baking tray with parchment paper.

3.   Roll the dough into balls (about a tablespoon each) and then roll in shredded coconut. Place on baking tray and place in fridge when all balls are formed.

4.   Chill at least 2 hours before serving.

Kiwi Lime Squares

Servings: Makes 10 squares

Total Time: 15 minutes plus 5 hours dehydrating time

Ingredients

- 1 cup raisins

- 1 cup almonds, soaked and drained

- 1 ½ cup dates

- 1/3 cup lime juice

- 1 kiwi, peeled and chopped

- 1 tablespoon lime zest

Directions

1.   Preheat oven to lowest available setting, preferably 100°F/40°C.

2.   Combine raisins and almonds in a food processor until a loose dough/crust texture forms. Press dough into a square 9" baking tray lined with parchment paper.

3.   Add dates, lime juice, kiwi and lime zest to blender and combine until smooth.

4.   Pour fruit mixture on top of crust and spread into even layer.

5.   Dehydrate in the oven for 5 hours before serving.

Chocolate Dipped Apricots

Servings: Makes 8 apricots

Total Time: 15 minutes plus 30 minutes chill time

Ingredients

- 2 tablespoons coconut oil, melted

- 1 tablespoon maple syrup

- 2 teaspoons raw cacao powder

- 8 apricot slices

- 1 tablespoon flaked sea salt

Directions

1. Line a baking tray with parchment paper.

2. In a small bowl, whisk together the coconut oil, maple syrup and cacao powder. Dip apricot slice halfway into the chocolate mixture.

3. Sprinkle sea salt on chocolate end of the apricot and place on baking tray.

4. Repeat with remaining 7 apricot slices and place tray in the fridge to chill for 30 minutes.

Raw Chocolate Donut Holes

Servings: 2

Total Time: 10 minutes plus 2 hours chilling

Ingredients

- ½ cup raw walnuts
- ½ cup raw almonds
- 10 dates, pitted and soaked 15 minutes then drained
- ½ tablespoon coconut oil
- ⅛ teaspoon Himalayan pink sea salt
- ¼ cup raw cacao powder
- ¼ teaspoon raw honey
- ½ teaspoon vanilla
- ¼ teaspoon ground cinnamon

Directions

1.   Add walnuts and almonds to the food processor and blend until finely ground.

2.   Add dates to nut mix and continue to process for about 2 minutes.

3.   Place remaining ingredients into the food processor and blend until combined and smooth.

4.   Roll dough into 1 tablespoon sized balls and chill in the fridge for at least 2 hours before serving.

Coconut Raspberry Bites

Servings: 2

Total Time: 10 minutes (optional 2 hours chilling)

Ingredients

- ½ cup almond meal
- 4 dates, pitted, soaked for 15 minutes then drained
- ½ cup unsweetened, shredded coconut, divided
- ¾ cup freeze-dried raspberries, divided
- ¼ cup cacao powder
- 3 tablespoons coconut butter, melted
- 3 tablespoons maple syrup
- 1 teaspoon vanilla extract
- ½ teaspoon Himalayan salt
- ¼ cup cacao nibs

Directions

1. Combine almond meal, dates, half of the shredded coconut, half of the raspberries, cacao powder, coconut butter, maple syrup, vanilla and salt in a food processor until smooth.

2.   Add in remaining coconut, raspberries and the cacao nibs. Pulse a few times so that these are incorporated but not entirely smooth.

3.   Roll dough into 1 tablespoon size balls.

4.   Either serve immediately or chill for 2 hours in the fridge before serving.

Double Chocolate Cookie Dough Bites

Servings: 2

Total Time: 10 minutes plus 2 hours chilling

Ingredients

- 1 cup oats

- 1 cup raw almonds

- ½ teaspoon salt

- ¼ teaspoon cinnamon

- 1 tablespoon vanilla extract

- 3 tablespoons maple syrup

- 2 tablespoons coconut oil, melted

- ¼ cup raw cacao powder

- ½ cup chickpeas, cooked

- 2 tablespoons cacao nibs

Directions

1.   In a food processor or high speed blender, add oats, almonds, salt, cinnamon and vanilla extract. Blend until a flour-like consistency is formed.

2.   Add in maple syrup, coconut oil, cacao and chickpeas. Blend until smooth and a dough forms.

3.   Stir in cacao nibs. Form into 1 tablespoon sized balls and chill for 2 hours before serving.

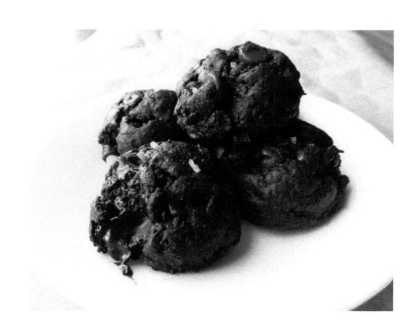

Veggie & Mango Sushi

Servings: 2 (1 sushi roll per serving)

Total Time: 35 minutes

Ingredients

- 2 nori sheets
- ½ zucchini, cut into thin strips
- 1 carrot, cut into thin strips
- 1 cup mango, cut into thin strips
- 1 cup sprouts
- 1 avocado, sliced

Cauliflower Rice

- ½ head cauliflower, cut into florets
- ½ tablespoon olive oil
- ½ cup quinoa, cooked and warmed
- ½ teaspoon tamari
- ½ teaspoon apple cider vinegar
- ½ teaspoon coconut aminos
- 1 teaspoon sesame seeds

Directions

1.   Process cauliflower florets in a food processor until a rice consistency is formed. Place cauliflower rice on a parchment paper lined baking tray, drizzle with olive oil and roast in an oven that has been preheated to 425°F/220°C for 25 minutes.

2.   Place roasted cauliflower and warm quinoa in a large bowl and add tamari, vinegar, coconut aminos and sesame seeds. Combine well until it becomes sticky and holds together slightly when pushed together.

3.   On a bamboo mat or tea towel in front of you, place a nori sheet and add half of the cauliflower rice at the end closest to you but leaving a slight space.

4.   Place half of the zucchini, carrot, mango, sprouts and avocado on top of the rice. Roll up starting with the edge closest to you and pressing in as you go.

5.   Repeat with the remaining nori, cauliflower rice and vegetables/fruit.

6.   Slice each roll into 8 pieces and serve.

Buddha Bowl

Servings: 2

Total Time: 35 minutes plus 5 hours in the fridge

Ingredients

- 1 bunch kale, stems removed and sliced into thin ribbons

- 1 tablespoon olive oil

- 1 teaspoon lemon juice

- 2 cups quinoa, cooked

- 1 cup lentils, cooked

- 10 cherry tomatoes, halved

- 1 zucchini, made into noodles with a spiralizer

- 1 avocado, sliced

- 1 tablespoon black sesame seeds

- 1 tablespoon green onions, thinly sliced

Tahini Dressing

- ¼ cup tahini

- ¼ cup warm water

- 1 teaspoon lemon juice

- 1 tablespoon maple syrup

- ½ teaspoon turmeric

- 1 garlic clove, minced

Pickled Radishes

- 3 red radishes, thinly sliced

- ¼ cup apple cider vinegar

- ¼ cup water

- 1 tablespoon honey

- 1 teaspoon Himalayan salt

- ½ jalapeno, seeded and diced

- 1 teaspoon whole black peppercorns

Directions

1.   In a jar that has a lid, place in all Pickled Radishes ingredients. Mix well and let sit for 5 hours in the fridge with the lid on. Make sure the radishes are always covered with liquid.

2.   Prepare Tahini Dressing by place all the ingredients in a small bowl and whisk together until smooth. If mixture is too thick, thin it out with more water.

3.   Place kale in a large mixing bowl and massage gently with the olive oil and lemon juice. Let rest 10 minutes.

4.   To assemble and serve, place kale at the bottom of a bowl and top with quinoa, lentils, tomatoes, zucchini noodles, avocado and pickled radishes. Drizzle with Tahini Dressing and sprinkle with black sesame seeds and green onions.

Confetti Cauliflower Rice

Servings: 2

Total Time: 20 minutes

Ingredients

- ½ cauliflower head, cut into florets

- 2 teaspoons olive oil

- 2 tablespoons red onion, chopped

- ¼ cup red bell pepper, chopped

- ¼ cup green bell pepper, chopped

- 1 garlic clove, minced

- 3 tablespoons water

- 1 teaspoon chili powder

- ¼ teaspoon ground cumin

- ½ teaspoon Himalayan salt

- ½ cup black beans

- ¼ cup cilantro, chopped

- 2 tablespoons green onions, thinly sliced

Directions

1.   Make cauliflower rice by processing the cauliflower florets in the food processor until it becomes a rice-like consistency.

2.   Heat olive oil in a medium skillet over medium-low heat. Add onion, red bell pepper, green bell pepper and garlic. Cook for 5 minutes before adding the cauliflower rice, water, chili powder, cumin and salt.

3.   Continue cooking another 5 minutes or until liquid is absorbed. Stir in black beans and cilantro and cook 2 minutes until warmed.

4.   Garnish with green onions and serve.

Creamy Sweet Salad

Servings: 2

Total Time: 20 minutes

Ingredients

- ½ teaspoon coriander powder

- ¼ teaspoon cumin

- ¼ teaspoon turmeric

- ¼ teaspoon cinnamon

- ½ teaspoon Himalayan salt

- ½ teaspoon black pepper, crushed

- 1 cup unsweetened yogurt

- 2 tablespoons olive oil

- 2 cups steamed brown rice

- 3 cups celery, sliced into ½ inch pieces

- 1 cup red bell pepper, diced

- 1 cup pear, cored, peeled and cut into 1 inch pieces

- 2 tablespoons green onions, thinly sliced

- 2 tablespoons raisins

- 1 tablespoon almonds, slivered

- 4 cups mixed greens

Directions

1.   In a small bowl, combine the coriander, cumin, turmeric, cinnamon, salt and pepper. Add to the yogurt and olive oil to the spice mixture. Let sit for 15 minutes.

2.   Place brown rice, celery, bell pepper, pear, green onions, raisins and almonds in a medium sized bowl. Pour yogurt mixture into the bowl and mix well to combine.

3.   Serve brown rice and pear mixture over mixed greens.

Sweet Spinach Salad

Servings: 2

Total Time: 15 minutes

Ingredients

- ¾ cup carrots, shredded
- 1 tablespoon lime juice
- ½ cup unsweetened yogurt
- ½ cup apple, cored and diced into 1 inch pieces
- ¼ cup raisins
- ¼ cup walnuts, toasted and chopped
- 2 tablespoons parsley, chopped
- 4 cups spinach, chopped
- 1 teaspoon cinnamon
- 1 teaspoon nutmeg
- 1 teaspoon Himalayan salt
- 1 teaspoon black pepper, crushed

Directions

1. Combine all ingredients in a large bowl and mix well.
2. Chill for 10 minutes before serving.

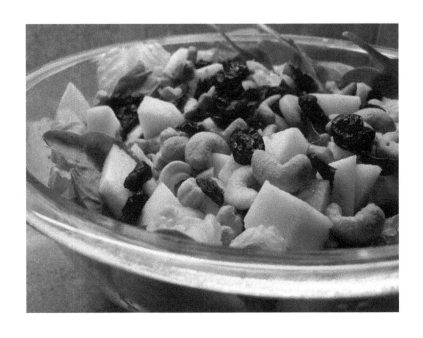

Green Hummus

Servings: 2

Total Time: 5 minutes

Ingredients

- 1 garlic clove
- 2 tablespoons green onion, sliced
- 1 cup chickpeas, drained and rinsed
- 2 tablespoons lemon juice
- ½ cup parsley, chopped
- 1 cup spinach, chopped
- 1 tablespoon cup tahini
- 2 tablespoons olive oil
- 2 tablespoons water
- 1 teaspoon cumin
- 1 teaspoon cayenne pepper
- ½ teaspoon Himalayan salt
- ¼ teaspoon black pepper
- 2 carrot, cut into sticks
- 2 celery stalks, trimmed and cut in half

Directions

1.   In a food processor or blender, combine all ingredients except the carrots and celery to create the hummus. Add more water if mixture is too thick.

Transfer to a small bowl and serve with carrots and celery.

Broccoli & Sprouts Savory Oats

Servings: 1

Total Time: 15 minutes

Ingredients

- 1 tablespoon olive oil
- 1 shallot, sliced
- 1 teaspoon nutritional yeast
- 1 teaspoon cayenne pepper
- ½ cup rolled oats
- ¾ cup unsweetened almond milk
- ¼ cup water
- 1 cup broccoli florets, steamed and chopped small
- ½ teaspoon Himalayan salt
- ½ teaspoon black pepper, crushed
- ½ cup alfalfa sprouts

Directions

1.	In a medium saucepan over medium heat add the oil, shallot, yeast and cayenne pepper. Cook 5 minutes and then add the oats, almond milk and water.

2.	Bring to a boil and reduce heat to low. Cook 5 minutes until liquid is absorbed.

3.	Stir in the broccoli, salt and pepper.

4.	Remove from heat and top with sprouts before serving

Fruit & Millet Breakfast

Servings: 2

Total Time: 30 minutes

Ingredients

- ½ cup millet
- 1 cup water
- 2 tablespoons raisins
- 1 tablespoon currants
- ⅛ teaspoon cinnamon
- ⅛ teaspoon vanilla extract
- 1 cup unsweetened coconut milk, divided
- 1 teaspoon honey
- ½ cup raspberries
- ½ cup blueberries
- 1 teaspoon hemp hearts
- 1 teaspoon chia seeds
- 1 teaspoon mint, chopped

Directions

1. Place millet and water in a medium saucepan over medium heat. Bring to a boil and then add the raisins, currants, cinnamon and vanilla. Cover with a lid, reduce heat to low and let cook for another 10 minutes until liquid is absorbed.

2. Turn heat off and let sit for 10 minutes

3. Add coconut milk, honey, raspberries, blueberries, hemp hearts and chia seeds. Turn heat to low and let cook for 2 minutes.

4. Transfer to bowls and garnish with mint.

Cheesy Bean Chips

Servings: 2

Total Time: 35 minutes

Ingredients

- 3 cups green beans
- ¼ cup avocado oil
- 2 teaspoon Himalayan salt
- ¼ cup nutritional yeast
- 1 teaspoon garlic powder
- 1 teaspoon onion powder
- 1 teaspoon paprika
- ½ teaspoon cayenne pepper

Directions

1.   Preheat oven to 400°F/205°C. Line a baking tray with parchment paper.

2.   Toss all ingredients in a medium-sized bowl to properly coat the green beans.

3. Place green beans on the baking tray and bake in the oven 30 minutes or until crispy.

Spinach & Artichoke Stuffed Mushroom

Servings: 2

Total Time: 20 minutes

Ingredients

- 6 white button mushrooms, stems removed and chopped (keep the remaining head of the mushroom)
- 1 cup spinach, steamed and chopped
- ¼ cup canned artichoke, drained and chopped
- ¼ cup nutritional yeast
- 1 tablespoon olive oil
- ¼ teaspoon garlic powder
- ¼ teaspoon onion
- ⅛ teaspoon pepper
- ¼ teaspoon Himalayan salt

Directions

1.   Add the mushroom stems, spinach, artichoke, nutritional yeast, olive oil, garlic, onion, pepper and salt to a food processor. Pulse a few times until combined but not entirely smooth.

2.   Preheat oven to 350°F/180°C and line a baking tray with parchment paper.

3.   Stuff each mushroom head with the spinach and artichoke mixture and place on the parchment paper.

4.   Bake for 15 minutes.

5.   Remove and serve hot.

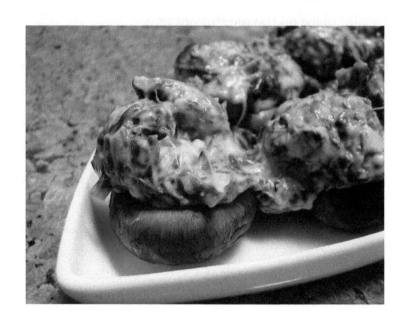

Quick Avocado Wraps

Servings: 2

Total Time: 5 minutes

Ingredients

- 4 Romaine lettuce leaves
- 1 avocado, sliced
- 1 ½ cups sprouts
- ½ cup hummus
- 1 cucumber, sliced
- 1 tablespoon sunflower seeds
- ¼ teaspoon Himalayan salt
- ¼ teaspoon black pepper, crushed

Directions

1. Stuff each lettuce leaf with the avocado, sprouts, hummus, cucumber, sunflower seeds, salt and pepper.

2. Roll up and enjoy.

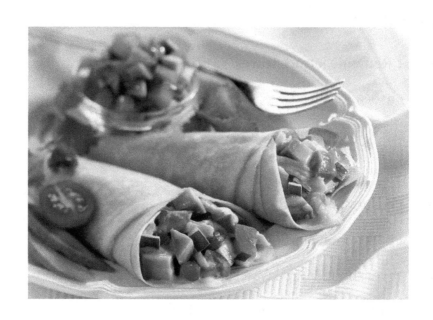

Strawberry Coconut Lime Bites

Servings: Makes 6 bites

Total Time: 10 minutes plus 30 minutes chill time

Ingredients

- 6 tablespoons unsweetened, shredded coconut
- 2 teaspoons lime zest
- ⅛ teaspoon Himalayan salt
- ¼ cup coconut butter, melted
- 6 strawberries

Directions

1. On a small plate, combine the shredded coconut, lime zest and salt

2. Take a small spoonful of the coconut butter and press it up against a strawberry. You may need to spread it around the strawberry with your fingers.

3. Roll the strawberry in the coconut lime mixture.

4. Repeat with the remaining strawberries.

5. Set on a large plate and chill in the fridge for at least 30 minutes before serving.

Coconut Chip Bites

Servings: Makes 8 bites

Total Time: 25 minutes

Ingredients

- 1 very ripe banana, mashed
- 2/3 cup unsweetened, shredded coconut
- 1 teaspoon coconut flour
- ¼ teaspoon vanilla extract
- ⅛ teaspoon Himalayan salt
- 1 teaspoon cacao nibs

Directions

1.   Preheat oven to 350°F/175°C. Line a baking tray with parchment paper.

2.   Combine all the ingredients in a large bowl. Mix thoroughly until dough-like texture is created.

3.   Spoon dough into 6 balls on the tray and press down on each ball.

4.   Bake in the oven for 10-15 minutes or until they are lightly browned.

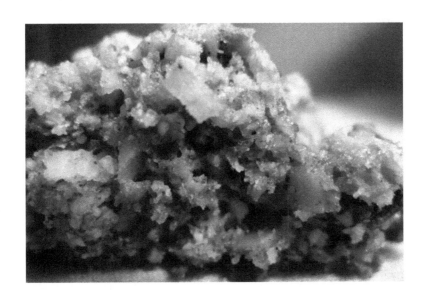

Sweet Potato Orange Cookies

Servings: Makes 12 cookies

Total Time: 35 minutes

Ingredients

- ¾ cup mashed sweet potato
- 1/3 cup quick oats
- 1 tablespoon cashew butter
- 1 egg
- 1 ½ tablespoon honey
- 1 teaspoon orange blossom water
- ¼ teaspoon vanilla
- ¼ teaspoon cinnamon
- ⅛ teaspoon nutmeg
- ¼ teaspoon baking powder
- ¼ teaspoon baking soda
- ⅛ teaspoon Himalayan salt
- 1 teaspoon orange zest
- 1 tablespoon raisins

Directions

1.   Preheat oven to 350°F/175°C. Line a baking tray with parchment paper.

2.   Add all the ingredients, except the raisins to a food processor and blend until combined. Fold in raisins.

3.   Scoop 12 balls of dough onto the baking tray. Flatten with a fork and bake for 20 minutes, flipping once halfway through.

4.   Remove and let cool before serving.

Strawberry Roll Ups

Servings: 2

Total Time: 5 minutes plus 4 hours cook time

Ingredients

- 1 cup strawberries, hulled and chopped
- ½ cup unsweetened applesauce
- 3 soft pitted dates

Directions

1. Preheat oven to 200°F/95°C. Line a baking tray with parchment paper.

2. Combine all the ingredients in a food processor or blender.

3. Pour the mixture onto the baking tray, spread it out into a thin layer and bake in the oven for 4 hours.

4. Remove and cut into strips to roll up

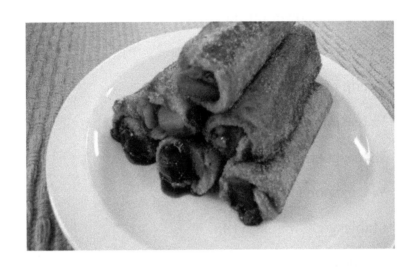

Pumpkin Pie & Cacao Fudge

Servings: 2

Total Time: 25 minutes plus 2 hours chill time

Ingredients

- ½ cup sunflower butter
- 2 tablespoons coconut oil
- ¼ cup pumpkin puree
- ½ teaspoon ground ginger
- ½ teaspoon ground cinnamon
- ¼ teaspoon ground nutmeg
- 1 tablespoon maple syrup
- 2 tablespoons cacao nibs

Directions

1. Line a small glass baking dish with parchment paper.

2. In a small saucepan over medium-low heat, melt sunflower butter and coconut oil. Stir in pumpkin puree, ginger, cinnamon, nutmeg and maple syrup. Keep occasionally stirring for about 15-20 minutes.

3. Remove from heat and fold in cacao nibs.

4.   Pour mixture into the baking dish and place in the fridge until firm, at least 2 hours.

Strawberry & Lime Balls

Servings: 2

Total Time: 5 minutes plus 30 minutes chill time

Ingredients

- 1/3 cup cashews
- ¾ cup shredded coconut
- ¼ cup diced strawberries
- 1 tablespoon maple syrup
- 1 lime, juiced
- 2 teaspoons lime zest
- 2 ½ tablespoons almond flour
- ½ teaspoon pure vanilla extract
- 2 tablespoons melted coconut oil

Directions

1.   Process the cashews in a food processor until a flour forms. Add the rest of the ingredients to the food processor and combine.

2.   Roll dough into small balls and place on a baking tray lined with parchment paper.

3.   Place in the freezer for at least 30 minutes before serving.

Papaya Popsicles

Servings: 2

Total Time: 5 minutes plus 4 hours freeze time

Ingredients

- ½ cup papaya, chopped

- ½ pineapple, chopped

- ¼ cup light coconut milk

- ½ cup coconut water

- 1 tablespoon raw honey

- 2 limes, zested and juiced

- 1 orange, juiced

Directions

1.   Combine all the ingredients in a blender and pour into popsicle molds.

2.   Place in the freezer for at least 4 hours.

Lemon Cashew Coated Strawberries

Servings: 2

Total Time: 10 minutes plus 1 hour chill time

Ingredients

- 1 cup raw cashews, soaked in cold water for 4 hours then drained and rinsed

- 1 cup pitted dates, pitted and soaked in cold water for 4 hours, drained and rinsed

- 1 tablespoon vanilla extract

- ¼ teaspoon almond extract

- 1 teaspoon lemon juice

- 1 teaspoon lemon zest

- ¼ teaspoon cinnamon

- 1 tablespoon unsweetened almond milk

- 1 pint of fresh strawberries, washed, dried, tops sliced off and middle scooped out

- 2 tablespoons mint, finely chopped

Directions

1.   In a food processor, combine the cashews, dates, vanilla, almond extract, lemon juice, lemon zest, cinnamon and almond milk until smooth.

2.   Spoon cashew mixture into each of the strawberries.

3.   Sprinkle mint on the top of the strawberry.

4.   Chill for 1 hour before serving.

Chai Tahini Ice Cream

Servings: 2

Total Time: 5 minutes plus 4 hours freeze time

Ingredients

- 1 can full fat coconut milk
- 1 tablespoon maple syrup
- ½ cup tahini
- ½ teaspoon ground cardamom
- ¼ teaspoon ground cinnamon
- ¼ teaspoon ground ginger
- ¼ teaspoon ground cloves

Directions

1. Place all the ingredients in a blender and mix until smooth.

2. Pour mixture into small, freezer-safe bowl and freeze at least 4 hours.

Apricot Crumble

Servings: 2

Total Time: 40 minutes

Ingredients

- 1 tablespoon coconut oil

- 5 apricots, coarsely chopped

- ½ cup raspberries

- 1 tablespoon chia seeds

- 1 tablespoon ginger, grated

- 1 tablespoon honey

- 1 cup rolled oats

- ½ cup ground almonds

- ¼ cup sliced almonds

- 1 tablespoon sunflower seeds

- ¼ cup unsweetened, shredded coconut

- ¼ cup maple syrup

- ¼ cup melted coconut oil

- ½ teaspoon salt

- ¼ teaspoon cinnamon

Directions

1.   Preheat oven to 350°F/175°C. Grease a small glass baking dish with 1 tablespoon of coconut oil.

2.   In a large bowl, combine the apricots and raspberries with the chia seeds, ginger and honey. Pour into the baking dish and set aside.

3.   Add the oats, ground almonds, sliced almonds, sunflower seeds, coconut, maple syrup, ¼ cup coconut oil, salt and cinnamon to the large bowl. Combine well so that entire mixture is moistened with the oil and syrup.

4.   Sprinkle oats mixture over the apricot and raspberry mixture.

5.   Bake in the oven for 30 minutes.

6.   Remove and let cool 5 minutes before serving.

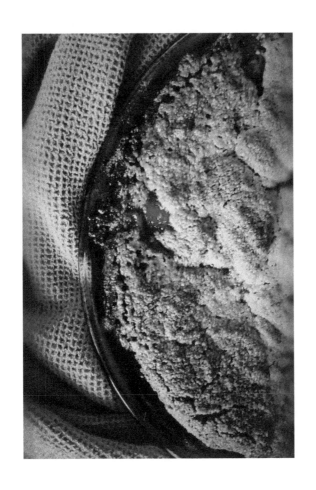

Lightning Source UK Ltd.
Milton Keynes UK
UKHW020619141222
413907UK00008B/72